How to Get Fat without Even Trying

"I am still amazed at how easy it was to get started, once I began reading Dana Pride's *How to Get Fat without Even Trying*. I didn't even finish the book and I already began to gain!" *–Dewayne A. Gainer*

"It's so simple, even a child can get fat by using just some of these techniques! Dana Pride has nailed a topic that previously has not had much attention." *–Getina Leddbottom*

"After trying just a few of these tips, I am on my way to obesity for life." *–Kent Seemytose*

"Although I have heard of some of these steps before, Dana Pride is the first to present the strategy that brings them all together." *–I. B. Round*

"Practical, useful information presented in an easy-to-understand way." *–Ima Snackin*

"I was surprised at how fast these techniques work, once I put them into my daily routine. The beauty of it is, I don't have to do all of them every day. Simply implementing one or two several times a week has already made a huge difference when I step on the scale. I just pick my favorites from the list and don't bother with the rest, and I am still seeing increased results!" *–Rayna de la Sayna*

"Gaining weight, gaining fat: what's the difference when you can do it so easily with Dana Pride's methods?" –*Will Eetitol*

"Even a flake can get fat using Dana Pride's simple strategies!" –*Dandrough Champeoux*

"The best part about this plan was that I didn't have to change my lifestyle and I can still eat all my favorite foods, as often as I want!" –*N. Joy Eaton*

"I am always skeptical of new suggestions on how to get fat, but this book tells you how to get results really fast! I am happy to announce, after only two weeks following just some of these ideas, I gained twelve pounds, and a month later, I have kept them on, plus, I have added seven more! This is a strategy I can use for life and will never have to worry about being thin again." –*Tippy da Scales*

How to Get Fat
without Even Trying

by
Dana Pride

Everlasting Publishing
Yakima, Washington
USA

How to Get Fat without Even Trying

by
Dana Pride

ISBN: 0-9852739-4-1
ISBN-13: 978-0-9852739-4-1

First Edition
Everlasting Publishing
P.O. Box 1061
Yakima, WA 98907

Thank you to Mom, Dad, my good friend, Farida, and to my husband for suggestions and encouragment while writing this book.

Dana

Warning: Following the suggestions in this book may lead to increased body mass. Increased body mass can cause backaches, sore knees, sore feet, sore ankles, upset stomach, diarrhea, constipation, headaches, increased risk of diabetes, increased risk of high cholesterol, increased risk of high blood pressure, increased risk of heart disease, the need for an entirely new wardrobe, decreased desire for sex, decreased desire to walk, inability to run or play sports, increased desire to watch television and increased desire to sit in front of the computer for hours without moving. Lack of movement can lead to muscle tension in the arms and shoulders, due to increased use of keyboard, computer mouse, remote control and video game controllers.

Many doctors will advise against the methods described in this book. Talk to your doctor before starting any fat-gaining program.

How to Get Fat without Even Trying

How to Get Fat without Even Trying

1.   Getting Started

You want to be above average, right? Who doesn't? In this decade, the average weight is much higher than it was 100 years ago, so you have to be consistently adding fat to stay above the rest.

What is fat? Who decides whether or not a person is fat? Does a person need to be a scientist or a doctor or have special knowledge in order to get fat and maintain the weight? How do we get fat? Can a person get fat fast, or does it take lots of time?

Fat is excess bulk on a person's body, a layer of cells under the skin. Regardless of a person's weight or height, he or she can have a small amount of fat or a large amount of fat on the body.

Society tends to be the contemporary judge who decides whether a person is fat or not fat. However, the scientific community today has published guidelines which suggest how much a person should weigh according to his or her height. Although in general these guidelines are accurate, a person can be considered 'overweight' and not have too much fat – if that weight is in excessive muscles. This book will not be covering that topic.

You, the general reader, can actually gain all the weight you want (and more!) without having any kind of degree or special training. If you follow the guidelines outlined in this book, I can (almost) guarantee that you will be on your way to obesity and beyond in a short amount of time. If you don't gain fat as rapidly as you desire, just stick with the program and you will gain in the long run.

A person gets fat by consistently consuming more calories than he or she burns. This book is not meant to be a scientific reference, but rather an easy, user-friendly guide to successfully adding fat to an individual body. I am not a doctor, but I have seen one on TV. You should consult your own doctor before attempting any of the processes listed in this book, if you want to get him on board with your fat-gaining plan.

You may be reading this book because you have long-term goals, such as having a good excuse not to go skiing or skating or biking or running or walking all over a golf course. Perhaps you see a future in which you don't have to walk, because you hope to get around in a electric scooter. Maybe you want people to feel sorry for you or ignore you completely, and by gaining a huge amount of fat, this will help you achieve those goals. Maybe you are a young person looking ahead to an early fat-related disability. The heavier you are, the more likely you are to achieve your fat-gain goals. Whatever your reason for reading this book, I thank you.

In this book, I use weight-gain and fat-gain interchangeably. Although a person can gain weight without gaining fat (by increasing muscle mass) the methods listed in this book will do nothing to add to your muscle mass or muscle weight. The weight you gain will be purely fat!

Please note: Results are typical for consistent users of the methods in this book.

2. Do Nothing

You may be one of the lucky ones, like I am, who can successfully gain weight and fat without doing anything! You may have a slow metabolism, you may have an underactive thyroid, you may be active or inactive, you may not pay any attention to what you are eating, and you are able to gain, gain, gain without doing a single thing to try to gain! Imagine that! You won't have to make any kind of change in your life! Who is comfortable with change? Don't we all want to remain in a personal comfort zone? You may be able to gain all you want and more, without doing anything.

Last year, in an 8-month period, I was able to put on one pound per month without even trying at all. I didn't do anything special. I didn't eat any more than usual, and I limited my desserts. I chose to eat what I considered to be healthy foods. I even started walking every day, and I was still able to faithfully gain a pound per month. I have experience in this area: I have been there.

You might be thinking, "Gain a pound per month? That's nothing! I can put on many more than that!" But can you, without trying? And if you want to do the math: adding one pound per month = 12 pounds per year = 120 pounds in 10 years. Between the ages of 30 and 50, you could successfully add 240 pounds to your weight! This means the average person who starts at 130 pounds could easily weigh 370 pounds twenty years later, without even trying.

If you are already over 50 years of age, you are probably saying, "I don't want to wait until I'm 70 to be that fat!" Guess what! The good news is, after the age of 50, your metabolism slows down, especially for women after menopause. This means you could easily be gaining two or three pounds per month, maybe even four or five, and you will be able to reach your fat-gain goals more quickly than you could when you were younger.

When I say "do nothing," I mean, literally, do nothing. You can take this in two ways: either don't do anything at all about your health and nutrition; or increase the time you spend doing nothing (sitting at your computer, sitting at your desk at work, sitting in front of the TV watching programs and movies or use your TV to play video games – the kinds of games that don't require standing and actively moving your body).

So, make sure you do NOT 'do the math.' Life is much easier when you don't have to think about addition, subtraction, and, especially, multiplication and division.

3. Pay No Attention

An easy way to gain weight is to pay no attention to what you eat, when you eat, where you eat, the amount of food you eat, or the kinds of foods you eat. Also, get rid of that scale! It will only serve to bug your conscience into controlling portions or feel guilty for enjoying all your favorite foods. Mindlessly eat whenever the mood strikes you. Keep your favorite snacks in the car, near the couch, in your desk drawers and in your pockets for easy access at any time.

Do you remember a song from the 1980s that included the phrase "you don't have to live your life in one day"? Forget that song! You can just go ahead to make it a point to eat all the food you love in one day and it will get you started on your way to weight-gain freedom! You won't gain muscle by just eating, but you can gain fat this way.

Whatever you do, do NOT look at the list of ingredients in the food you buy. Focus on packaged and pre-made meals when you are shopping at the grocery store. Keep your eyes on the supermarket shelves at eye-level, since that is where the most popular foods are presented. Don't bother looking up high or down low on the shelves; that's where they put the foods for people who want to eat unpopular food or the cheaper store brands.

On a final note in not paying attention, make sure you do not measure your serving sizes. Just serve yourself what you consider to be a healthy portion, and it will almost always be more than your body needs to maintain your weight.

4.   If You Do Pay Attention…

Are you one of those obsessive-compulsive types who has to pay attention to everything you do? Maybe you like to think about everything you eat. I am not telling you to step out of your comfort zone and stop paying attention. After all, this book is all about sliding into your comfort zone and staying there.

You can still get fat even if you pay attention to what you are eating, drinking and doing. This chapter focuses on specific things that can help you achieve your fat-gaining goals, without just 'letting it happen' naturally, without thought.

a. Snack yourself fat (between-meal boost)

You can easily gain pounds here, there and everywhere by snacking! Those added calories between meals may not seem to be making a difference, but in time, they will.

Are you snacking enough?

- Do you have a large bowl of your favorite bite-size candy beside your computer, and another one by your TV-watching chair or couch?

- Do you have at least one cupboard in your kitchen full of crackers, candy, cookies, chips and nuts? Yes, I mention nuts, because in large quantities, they are both healthy and fattening. You want to make sure you have plenty of foods available that need no preparation so you can often grab a handful without thinking and pop it in your mouth.

- Do you have lots of your favorite non-melting snacks handy in your car, for those short or long trips when you can save time by eating and driving simultaneously?

You don't actually need to waste time or thought measuring or pouring your chips or cookies into a bowl. Simply take the entire bag or box to the couch or computer so you won't have to return to the kitchen unnecessarily for refills.

Remember when your mother used to tell you to not snack between meals because it will spoil your appetite? This simply is not true! You will get another appetite, and as your body gets used to the variety of snacks between meals, you can actually train yourself to feel hungry more often!

b.   Get to the fast food joint fast!
     (drive thru to your favorite flavors)

What is quicker and easier than getting fast food through the drive-thru? With fast food, you spend no time planning, shopping, preparing and cooking. You don't even have to spend time rearranging food on your refrigerator shelves to fit in something new. At the drive-thru window, you are able to get exactly what you feel like eating, right at that very moment!

I don't live in a large city, but even in my town, we have an abundance of fast food available and we are able to stay in the car to get it. Some of the always-ready choices, besides a huge range of the favorite hamburger and fries, are: chicken (regular, crispy or spicy), pizza (thick or thin crust), chili dogs (with or without beans), tacos (small and enormous), burritos (plain or stuffed with just about anything) and sub sandwiches (half-foot, one foot and longer)! Compliment your main course with chunky side dishes and satisfying supply of soda pop in a 44-ounce cup and you might stay full for at least an hour or two.

Often just one fast food meal will include enough calories and fat for your entire day, so everything you eat besides that meal will easily be adding to your fat-gain process. Don't bother wasting time and energy getting out of your car when you can do it the easy way and drive-thru to meals at least once every day.

Don't forget your well-deserved favorite dessert! Many drive-thru restaurants offer the standard ice cream cone, sundae and milkshake. Now you can also get a conglomeration of multi-flavored ice cream, cookies, candies and toppings mixed into your sundaes and shakes. For most places, you don't need to find a coupon from the newspaper or a magazine: if you go often enough, you may be eligible to get a frequent buyer's discount!

c. Eat larger meals
    (buy bigger plates)

In order to avoid having to return to the stove or refrigerator for seconds and thirds, buy some larger plates so you can load up one time! Many of us are programmed to eat the amount of food before us on our plate – it's only polite, isn't it, to eat all of our food? We don't want to waste any food, because people in some other country are starving. As your stomach stretches, you won't notice the larger portions, and you will be eating your way to your potential fat person by bigger meals alone!

Use the same concept at restaurants:

- Buy the largest portion of your main dish.

- Add the largest available size of side dishes (and be sure to NOT select vegetables!)

- You can often add more side dishes at a discount – save money!

- If you don't see the larger portion meal on the menu, just ask! Restaurants are in the business of pleasing customers, and they will usually accommodate you.

17

- Don't save any of your meal for later. It tastes best when you eat it all at the restaurant.

Buy in bulk! You save money that way, and you will be sure to always have your favorite frozen food, boxed food and snacks on hand. Why wait to enjoy the food you love, when you can have access to it any time?

When you settle in for your nightly bowl of ice cream covered with chocolate, caramel and/or hot fudge, use a serving bowl. Eat buttery popcorn from the largest mixing bowl you have in the kitchen. Save your salad bowls for lettuce or any type of food you intend to minimize during your fat-gain journey.

As for sandwich-making, the taller, the better! Use the large size bread, plenty of mayonnaise, and stacks of cheese and meat to make it as tall as possible while still being able to squish it to fit into your mouth. Have fun with your sandwich! Be creative, by layering the cheese and meat into a colorful striped stack. You will be proud of the inspiration you can get by making the tallest, most colorful sandwich you have ever seen. Feel free to send me a picture of your creations – before you eat them, obviously.

d. Add a late-night meal
   (convert snack to meal)

Do you get hungry late at night? Who made the rule that three large meals per day are enough, anyway? You can easily add another meal to your daily routine and soon your body will let you know that it's time for that fourth meal of pizza or those tacos or another roast beef sandwich and bag of potato chips. No matter in what region of the country you live, you can enjoy breakfast, lunch, dinner AND supper!

You don't have to do the math, but you will easily be adding 25-33% more calories to your daily intake with this method. Your rapidly growing body will show you, your family and the world that three meals per day don't have to be the standard, when you can easily eat four! After practicing this for just one week, I can almost guarantee that your stomach will be growling late at night, begging you to fill it one more time with another meal (not just snacks).

e. More carbs
    (less protein)

Carbohydrates are the joy of life! If you are not sure what a carbohydrate is, or 'carb,' as it is fondly known, don't worry! Most of the foods you love are carbohydrates.

These are the yummy foods that you should be eating most often so you can more rapidly increase your weight. Don't grab protein (meat, beans, eggs, fish) unless you eat it with a large amount of carbs, since protein will keep you feeling full.

One way to be sure you get your carb quota when you do eat protein is to select protein sources that are coated and deep fried: chicken strips, chicken fingers, breaded chicken patties, breaded fish, fish sticks, and deep fried shrimp, to name a few.

Have you ever noticed that eating something sweet early in the day makes you crave sweets all day long? This is a great way to go from sweet to sweet! Start your day with a few donuts, which I like to call tripple-whammies, since they are made of white flour, full of sugar, and deep fried. They are just so yummy! They'll start your yearning for more sweets.

Also, in some people, eating sweets triggers the urge to eat something salty, making a nice transition, sweet-salty-sweet-salty. Either way your cravings take you, this can help you achieve your fat-gain goals much more quickly than avoiding these foods completely.

Carbs include:

- Cookies

- Crackers

- Chips

- Candy

- Cakes

- Cereal

- Donuts

- Bread

- Fruit

- Vegetables (Be sure to choose vegetables that have become high-calorie foods: deep fried vegetables, such as fried potatoes, fried onion rings, fried mushrooms, fried zucchini. If you do select salads, slather them with a large portion of high-fat dressing.)

f.   Don't Choose
      (let someone else decide what you eat)

Who decides what you are going to put in your mouth?

Those of you who live alone, you may think that you alone are making all your food decisions. However, you are easily influenced by advertisements in magazines and on the Internet, as well as television commercials. Do not plan ahead. Planning your meals in advance may cause you to think about what you are eating and try to balance your calorie intake. Just go with the flow and take your suggestions from your persuasive environment. Doesn't a nice, thick slice of pizza dripping with cheese sound good right now, along with a liter of soda pop?

If you are living in a family situation, you will find it much easier to let someone else decide what you are going to eat. If you are not the one who cooks most of the meals or buys most of the food, you can simply eat what is placed before you. In order to increase the amount of fat on your body in this situation, just eat more (see subchapters 4b and 4c).

If you happen to be the one who makes the food decisions in your family, you can make sure your entire family gets larger along with you. You won't be gaining alone, as long as you follow the methods in this book. Be sure to have those extra portions available at meal time, as well as keeping the cupboards stocked with the snacks your family loves the most. When you go shopping, buy two or three large packages instead of a small one, so you won't deprive any family members of something at the moment they want it. They want it now! You, like the person who lives alone, can also be influenced by advertisements and commercials, so pay particular attention to them at all times!

g. Buy multi-ingredient items

This tip is only for people who choose to read the labels on their packaged food. If you don't want to bother with reading labels, skip ahead to the next chapter.

On package labels, more is better when it comes to ingredients and fat-gain. If you are reading a nice, long list of ingredients in a product and you come across something you can't pronounce or don't know what it is, that is something you want to put into your mouth to help enlarge your body! Look for the words 'hydrogenated' and 'modified,' two completely unnatural ingredients. Added fat in products translates to added fat on your body.

If you add enough unnatural or unknown ingredients to your daily intake, you will see a gradual increase when you step on the scale. This method is not always the fastest way to get fat, so you will probably want to use this one in conjunction with another method listed in this book in order to see large changes in your body more quickly.

5.   Not the Water, but a Lot More!

Your liquid intake can greatly add to your calorie numbers, and you won't even feel any fuller than if you were just drinking water! My suggestion for those who need hundreds of extra calories every day is to drink plenty of sugary drinks all day long.

Start your morning with one of those flavored coffees from a drive-thru coffee stop. If you are one of the rare persons who doesn't like coffee, most places offer all kinds of chocolate drinks and flavored drinks, hot or cold. For an early morning calorie boost, try the largest size chocolate-mocha extra sweet with a double shot of flavoring. Depending on how large is the large, you may be starting your day with an extra 800-1000 calories – but who's counting? Certainly you aren't! A better idea is to purchase one of those large mugs that holds at least 42 ounces and then you only are paying for the refill. Most coffee places give you a discount when you bring your own cup!

During the day, be sure to keep your sugary drinks nearby. If you are an all-day coffee drinker, keep your canister of sugar at your desk or worksite so you can make sure to stay sweetened throughout the day.

Another good option to help with gaining is soda pop. Did you know you can actually save money by buying lots of soda pop? For instance, look at any vending machine that sells both pop and water. The cost of the pop is normally 75 cents while water is $1.25. For those who are mathematically challenged, this means ten trips to the vending machine can save you $5.00 if you only buy soda pop and not water! That's $5.00 every work week, if you visit the vending machine twice per day!

Forget the small stuff. You can find two liters (roughly a half gallon) of soda pop on sale for 79 cents or 99 cents just about any time of the year. Believe it or not, adding just one two-liter bottle of soda pop to your diet per day can easily add 30-40 pounds per year onto your weight! You won't need to make any type of lifestyle changes and you don't have to do the math. You can continue living the same way as you are living today and just this one simple change will rapidly increase your size, without weighing you down with added muscle.

Don't even consider drinking plain water. Drinking water tends to make you feel full, and that can deter you from wanting that extra snack or that large meal – or even your newly-established late-night meal (see subchapter 4c). Our bodies are made up of mostly water. Why would you want to merely add more water to your body?

6.   Sit Still!

It's a scientific fact: objects at rest tend to stay at rest (until pushed). Don't push yourself! Enjoy the sitting as long as you can! Walking and moving about, even standing up from the chair, use some calories, and that is what you do NOT want to do when you are in a weight-gaining mode.

Are you familiar with the law of gravity? When an object sits still for a long enough time, molecules begin to settle down – at the bottom. When you sit still for a long enough time, over time, you begin to see an enlarging of the area of gravitational pull – your bottom.

However, you don't have to be a scientist to enjoy the gaining of fat! Just sit back and relax, and it will eventually happen.

7. Stay Awake

In order to help the suggestions in the other chapters to work at their best, make sure you don't get enough sleep. Better yet, while staying up late to watch your favorite after-hours programming, have that fourth or fifth meal or that second dessert (see subchapter 4d). I can assure you that the commercials on television will trigger your appetite late into the night, when you might otherwise be sleeping.

Getting fewer than 7 hours of sleep per night will surely be a benefit to anyone who is trying to pack on the pounds. This can help in a couple of ways. When you are feeling tired during the day, you won't want to be active. You will feel like sitting or relaxing at work or at home all day long. You will have no ambition to walk or ride your bike, and you especially won't want to go all the way to the gym. Most likely, you will be inclined to recline, since lack of a good night's sleep will leave you with a lack of energy.

Another fat-gaining benefit of not getting enough sleep: Have you noticed that when you are feeling groggy at work (or at home when you don't have time to take a nap), a sweet snack can do something to help revive you? This is the time you can look forward to some of those really handy treats that require no preparation. Why wait 30 seconds for a hot dog in the microwave when you can pop a handful of candy in your mouth immediately? Be sure to keep giant cookies on hand, since they serve dual purpose: they are easy to eat and they make you feel like you are eating enough.

8. Add Stress

Until recently, stress has not been associated with weight gain. However, studies have now shown that a nice dose of stress in your life can lead to unconscious eating, mindless snacking, reduction of restful sleep and a larger you! Adding stress can also help cut down on your restful sleep, which can also help you gain fat without trying (see Chapter 7).

Is your life too peaceful? Is your job a piece of cake? (Why don't you enjoy a piece of cake right now, while reading this?) Are you living below your possible stress level?

Here are some things to think about that may help to add stress that can help you get fat:

- You are not as successful as _____ (Fill in the blank with your neighbor, your brother, your parents, your classmates, a software billionaire.)

- You, or someone in your family, could be diagnosed with a deadly disease.

- You could be in a disabling accident tomorrow – or even today!

- A tornado could hit your town.

- A volcano could erupt near your town.

- Alligators could come to your door and not let you out of the house.

- You could get audited by just about anyone for just about anything.

- You could be blamed for something you didn't do.

- People could discover your secret.

- You could lose all your money.

- Your favorite program will probably be cancelled.

- You may lose your Internet connection.

- Someone might steal your identity.

- If you have a job, you could lose it.

- If you don't have a job, you could be forced to get one.

- You might not get enough sleep tonight.

If nothing on this list triggers enough stress, send me an email and I'll send you an in-depth list of Things that Could Possibly Happen to Make Your Life Worse (therefore adding stress.)

9. Maintaining Your Greater Weight

You may be worried that once you achieve your greater weight goal, you won't be able to maintain it. You might be afraid that the pounds will mysteriously disappear while you sleep, without you doing anything to create a loss of weight.

No need to worry, my friend! As long as you continue doing even some of the things I have mentioned in this book, you won't lose more than a few pounds. As a matter of fact, if you do lose a little bit of weight, don't fret about it. You can easily regain those missing pounds and add a few more by snacking (subchapter 4a), drinking sugary drinks (chapter 5), enlarging your portions (subchapter 4c) and slowing down your body movement (chapter 6).

Above all, here are the three things to NOT do:

- Exercise

- Portion what you eat

- Load up on mainly vegetables

You will find it to be so easy to maintain your greater weight, pretty soon you won't have to think about it --ever!

10.   Larger for Life & Quick Tips

A person doesn't have to be a mathematician or a scientist in order for these mathematic and scientific principles to work on the body to increase fat. By following some or all of the suggestions listed in this book, even the ordinary person can get fat without even trying.

Unless you have some strange disease that prevents you from getting fat, I can guarantee that if you consistently follow only half of the strategies listed in this book, you will get fat. Don't expect an overnight change, but stick with the methods and you will be satisfied with your gradually-forming rotund shape.

Fat people are jolly, aren't they? You can join the jolly and it will happen more quickly than you expect! Your jeans will grow tight and become impossible to fasten. You will no longer be able to button your shirt and coat. You will have an excuse to get a whole new wardrobe! Before you know it, you will be shopping in the King and Queen sizes, checking to see if the clothes you like are X or XX or 3X or 4X. You will actually be able to fill a mu-mu!

As I mentioned at the beginning of the book, I began on this path of gaining and I gradually saw progress. The only reason I am not even fatter than I was just a year ago is because I was not consistent in using these methods. I paid attention to ingredients and portion sizes. I stopped drinking all sugary drinks and switched to drinking lots of water every day. I increased the amount of exercise I was doing. I removed snacks from my home, my office and my car, and I began to plan my meals. However, this was probably my biggest fat-killer: I stopped eating when I was pleasantly full.

When you see my photo and wonder why I am not my own poster child for fatness, just remember: I am not following my own advice.

In summary, here are some Quick Tips to getting fat. Remember, the more you follow, the more quickly you will see large results!

1. Take it easy! Don't plan, don't read, don't exercise, don't worry!

2. Treat yourself – every day! You deserve to have whatever you want, whenever you want, so help yourself to that treat that you are craving!

3. Load your liquids! Stay away from plain water and drink the most flavorful drinks you desire – often.

4. Save some money! Cancel your gym membership, sell your bike, sell your skis, don't buy ski tickets, sell your golf clubs, sell your skates, sell your home exercise equipment, and get some money back on those things you bought but will never use.

5. Keep it handy! Put your favorite snacks – especially the bite-size goodies – well within reach: near your couch, near your desk, in your car, by your bed. You never know when you may have an impulse to munch on some chocolate chunks or a salty snack, so be sure you don't have to go far to get it.

Most of all, enjoy your new freedom to eat, eat, eat, all you want, whatever you want, all the time!

You may think, after reading this book, that it is a joke. However, I have never been more serious in my life than I am right now. If you honestly follow the strategies I have listed, you will very soon be able to gain weight without even thinking about it. When you look in the mirror, you will soon see a lot more of yourself.

Dana Pride

AFTER THE GREAT DEVASTATION

a novel by Dana Pride

A global disaster, known as The Great Devastation, drastically changed life on earth. Layla, a Kidgen, or Kid-Genius, is living and working at the Complex, where the Insiders have everything they need provided for them: jobs, food, clothing, entertainment. Layla is aware of the Outsiders, (the Ordinaries, the Crims, the Chairs and the Runners) who are just scraping by without the use of technology, but she doesn't have any reason to think much about them - until Kenrick, one of her friends who is also a Kidgen and a Comgen (Computer-Genius), secretly arranges for four friends to travel.

Suddenly Layla becomes curious. What is life Outside really like? Where will they go? What will they eat? Will they be able to get back safely and unpunished? Kenrick has a few surprises in store for them, especially for Layla, whose life will never be the same after they make their journey outside the Complex.

COMING SOON!
Book 2: The Hidden City

www.ingramcontent.com/pod-product-compliance
Lightning Source LLC
Chambersburg PA
CBHW071412200326
41520CB00014B/3407